FACELIFT SURGERY NUTRITION PLAN

Comprehensive Guide Unlocking The Secrets of nutrition after Surgery Success, Nourishing Meal Plans, Recipes And Practical Tips For Optimal Health And Wellness)

DR. ALLAN FREDA

Contents

1. Expert advice: After undergoing a facelift, the book provides expert advice on how to create a diet plan that will help the body recuperate. This advice is based on tried-and-true tactics that nutritionists and doctors have suggested.

2. Recipes for Healing: This section offers readers a variety of recipes that are designed to supply vital vitamins, minerals, and nutrients for the best possible recovery. These recipes have been thoughtfully created to improve general wellness, lessen inflammation, and encourage healing.

3. Meal Plans: The book offers individualized meal plans that are designed to satisfy each person's specific nutritional requirements following facelift surgery. These meal plans are designed to provide a well-rounded and nutritional diet during the recuperation phase, taking into consideration dietary preferences, constraints, and requirements.

4. Long-Term Wellness: The book stresses the significance of long-term wellness in addition to the acute post-surgery diet. To promote prolonged health and vigor, readers will learn ways to keep up a good diet and lifestyle after the recovery phase.

OVERVIEW

Recognizing the Relationship Between Diet and Facelift Surgery:

Rhytidectomy, another name for facelift surgery, is a cosmetic technique that aims to rejuvenate the face by minimizing aging indicators including wrinkles and drooping skin. It is impossible to overestimate the significance of diet in the pre-and post-operative stages, even while the surgery itself plays a big part in attaining the intended aesthetic result. A person's diet is fundamental to their general health and well-being, and it has a significant effect on the results of surgeries, particularly facelift procedures.

Before getting into the details of a diet designed specifically for facelift surgery, it is important to comprehend the physiological mechanisms underlying the procedure as well as the body's healing response. Incisions are made, facial tissues are lifted and repositioned, and extra skin may be removed during a facelift procedure. In addition to improving looks, these operations cause stress to the body, which sets off an inflammatory reaction and starts the healing process.

The fundamental components and nutrients required for tissue repair, collagen formation, and general recovery are provided by a healthy diet.

Moreover, a balanced diet has advantages that go beyond wound healing. To avoid infections, boost the immune system, and reduce inflammation—all critical components of the post-surgery recovery process—nutrients are essential. Sufficient diet can also reduce the chance of problems, hasten recovery, and improve appearance.

Thus, creating a thorough nutrition plan that is customized to each patient's needs after facelift surgery is essential to encouraging the best possible results and guaranteeing long-term health.

A Complete Guide To The Best Post-Surgery Diet, Including Healing Recipes, Meal Plans, And Professional Advice For Long-Term Wellness, For Those Just Diagnosed:

It can be difficult to navigate the recovery after surgery, particularly with food choices. With this extensive book, we hope to give newly diagnosed patients having facelift surgery a road map to healthy nutrition, complete with therapeutic recipes, adaptable meal plans, and professional advice for long-term wellness. Through a comprehensive dietary approach that emphasizes nutrient-dense foods, supplementing when needed, and prioritizing water, people can facilitate their bodies' natural healing processes and see long-lasting benefits.

Remedy Recipes:

The post-surgery diet is incomplete without healing dishes, which provide nutritional and easily digestible options that aid in the healing and recovery process. With nutrient-dense components like whole grains, fruits, vegetables, lean proteins, and healthy fats, these dishes offer the building blocks needed for tissue regeneration and repair. Furthermore, some components—like turmeric, ginger, and leafy greens—that are well-known for their anti-inflammatory and antioxidant qualities can aid in lowering the swelling, bruising, and inflammation that are frequently connected to facelift surgery.

Meal Schedules:

Meal plans that are adaptable to each person's dietary requirements and tastes are a useful tool for making sure that a balanced diet is followed during the healing process. Taking into consideration particular dietary limitations or preferences, these meal plans include meals and snacks for breakfast, lunch, supper, and snacking. People can successfully support their bodies' healing processes and maximize their nutritional intake by including a variety of nutrient-dense foods and maintaining a balance of macronutrients. Additionally, by taking the uncertainty out of meal preparation, meal planning can reduce stress and make the recovery process after surgery easier.

Professional Advice for Long-Term Health:

Adding professional advice for long-term well-being is crucial to preserving the advantages of facelift surgery and enhancing general health and vigor, in addition to healing recipes and eating regimens.

To promote the best possible healing and cosmetic results, these suggestions may include advice on hydration, supplements, skincare, stress management, and lifestyle adjustments.

For instance, maintaining proper hydration is essential for encouraging tissue hydration, eliminating toxins, and assisting in cellular regeneration and repair. Similarly, adding supplements like collagen, zinc, and vitamin C may improve skin health and speed up the healing of wounds.

Furthermore, maintaining the outcomes of facelift surgery and promoting skin regeneration can be achieved by establishing a regular skincare regimen utilizing mild, non-irritating products. It's also critical to manage stress through mindfulness exercises, relaxation techniques, and enough sleep to maximize healing and promote general well-being. Last but not least, leading a healthy lifestyle that includes consistent exercise, a well-balanced diet, and mindful eating practices will help maintain long-term wellness and guarantee that results from facelift surgery last.

after facelift surgery, a thorough dietary plan is critical to maximizing recovery and fostering long-term wellness.

People may assist their bodies' healing processes and achieve long-lasting results by learning the link between nutrition and surgery outcomes, adding healing recipes, creating customisable meal plans, and getting expert advice for long-term wellness. People can improve their general health and energy, preserve the benefits of facelift surgery, and accelerate their recovery with a holistic approach to diet and lifestyle.

Disclaimer

The information in this book is for informational purposes only and should not replace professional medical advice, diagnosis, or treatment. Always consult your physician or a qualified health provider regarding any medical concerns. Do not disregard professional medical advice or delay seeking it based on information in this book.

The author does not endorse or have affiliations with any mentioned entities. References are for informational purposes only.

Consult your healthcare provider before making dietary or lifestyle changes, especially during recovery from surgery, as individual needs vary.

Results may vary, and the information provided is not guaranteed to produce specific outcomes.

By reading this book, you acknowledge and agree to consult your healthcare provider before implementing any information herein.

For further guidance, consult your healthcare provider or reputable medical websites for reliable information on surgery recovery diets.

CHAPTER 1
PRE-SURGERY PREPARATION

To maximize results and encourage healing, facelift surgery—a common cosmetic operation meant to rejuvenate the facial appearance—requires meticulous pre-operative preparation.

A vital component of this preparation is making sure the body gets enough nourishment from foods high in nutrients. An important part of boosting the body's immune system, improving wound healing, lowering inflammation, and lowering the chance of problems is eating a healthy diet before surgery.

As a result, individuals having facelift surgery should concentrate on eating a diet that is well-balanced and rich in protein, vitamins, minerals, and antioxidants.

The significance of loading your body with foods high in nutrients:

As part of the pre-operative preparation phase, the diet must be given top priority before facelift surgery. Eating a diet high in nutrients fortifies the immune system of the body, which is essential and boosts warding off infections and facilitating speedy healing following surgery. Essential vitamins including vitamin C, vitamin E, and vitamin A are found in nutrient-rich meals and are important for the creation of collagen, tissue healing, and overall skin health. Minerals that promote wound healing and immune system function include zinc and selenium.

Moreover, adding antioxidants to the diet can aid in lowering inflammation and oxidative stress, two frequent reactions to surgery. Fruits, vegetables, nuts, and seeds are good sources of antioxidants, which work to scavenge free radicals and shield cells from harm. This is especially crucial when it comes to facelift surgery since it can lessen tissue damage and facilitate a more comfortable recovery.

For tissue regeneration and repair, a sufficient protein intake is necessary in addition to vitamins, minerals, and antioxidants. Lean meats, chicken, fish, eggs, dairy products, legumes, and tofu are examples of foods high in protein that supply the building blocks needed for the production of new tissue and collagen, both of which are essential for getting the best possible outcomes following facelift surgery.

Recipes for Detoxification and Pre-Surgery Cleaning:

Patients may think about including detoxification and cleansing recipes in their diet as part of their pre-surgery preparation to aid in the removal of toxins, lower inflammation, and promote general health and well-being. These recipes frequently call for foods like citrus fruits, leafy greens, cruciferous vegetables, and fresh herbs that are well-known for their purifying qualities.

A green detox smoothie composed of spinach, kale, cucumber, celery, green apple, lemon juice, and ginger is an illustration of a purifying recipe.

This nutrient-dense smoothie is a great option for pre-surgery sustenance because it is high in vitamins, minerals, and antioxidants. In order to get the body ready for the impending surgery, it supports liver function, aids in detoxification, and alkalizes the body.

Detoxifying vegetable soup, prepared with a range of vibrant veggies including carrots, bell peppers, tomatoes, onions, garlic, and herbs like cilantro and turmeric, is another alternative for cleansing.

This tasty soup is a great addition to the pre-surgery diet since it is full of minerals and phytonutrients that help the body's detoxification pathways, increase immunity, and reduce inflammation.

Incorporating these cleansing and detoxifying recipes into the pre-surgery nutrition plan can help optimize the body's internal environment, enhance the body's ability to heal, and support overall health and well-being before undergoing facelift surgery. However, it is essential to consult with a healthcare professional or a registered dietitian before making any significant dietary changes, especially before surgery, to ensure that individual nutritional needs and medical considerations are taken into account.

CHAPTER 2

POST-SURGERY RECOVERY NUTRITION

Facelift surgery is a significant procedure that requires careful attention not only during the operation but also in the post-operative phase. Proper nutrition plays a crucial role in facilitating optimal healing and recovery after facelift surgery. In this comprehensive guide, we will delve into the nutritional needs during the initial recovery phase, explore soft foods and liquid diets that aid healing, and discuss anti-inflammatory recipes aimed at reducing swelling and bruising post-surgery.

Nutritional Needs During the Initial Recovery Phase

Following facelift surgery, the body undergoes a period of healing and regeneration. During this time, it is essential to provide the body with adequate nutrients to support tissue repair, reduce inflammation, and boost the immune system.

Protein is particularly important during the initial recovery phase as it provides the building blocks necessary for tissue repair and regeneration. Incorporating lean protein sources such as chicken, fish, tofu, and legumes into meals can help promote healing and accelerate recovery. Additionally, vitamins and minerals such as vitamin C, vitamin A, zinc, and omega-3 fatty acids play key roles in the healing process and should be included in the post-surgery diet. Fruits, vegetables, nuts, and seeds are excellent sources of these essential nutrients and should be consumed regularly to support optimal recovery.

Soft Foods and Liquid Diets to Aid Healing

During the early stages of recovery following facelift surgery, patients may experience difficulty chewing and swallowing due to swelling and discomfort. In such cases, incorporating soft foods and liquid diets into the post-surgery nutrition plan can help ease these challenges while providing essential nutrients to support healing.

Soft foods such as mashed potatoes, yogurt, smoothies, and soups are easy to consume and gentle on the digestive system, making them ideal choices for individuals recovering from surgery. Additionally, incorporating nutrient-dense liquids such as protein shakes, vegetable juices, and bone broth into the diet can help maintain hydration and provide essential vitamins and minerals necessary for healing. It is essential to consult with a healthcare professional or registered dietitian to develop a personalized nutrition plan tailored to individual needs and preferences during the recovery phase.

Anti-Inflammatory Recipes for Reduced Swelling and Bruising

Swelling and bruising are common side effects of facelift surgery and can prolong the recovery process if not managed effectively. Fortunately, incorporating anti-inflammatory foods into the post-surgery diet can help reduce swelling, bruising, and discomfort, promoting faster healing and recovery.

Including foods rich in antioxidants such as berries, leafy greens, and citrus fruits can help neutralize free radicals and reduce inflammation in the body. Turmeric, ginger, and garlic are potent anti-inflammatory spices that can be incorporated into recipes to further enhance their healing properties.

Additionally, omega-3 fatty acids found in fatty fish, flaxseeds, and walnuts have been shown to have anti-inflammatory effects and may help alleviate swelling and bruising post-surgery.

By focusing on a diet rich in anti-inflammatory foods and incorporating healing recipes into meals, individuals can support the body's natural healing processes and optimize recovery following facelift surgery.

proper nutrition is essential for optimal healing and recovery following facelift surgery.

By understanding the nutritional needs during the initial recovery phase, incorporating soft foods and liquid diets to aid healing, and including anti-inflammatory recipes in the post-surgery nutrition plan, individuals can support their bodies natural healing processes and promote long-term wellness. It is crucial to consult with a healthcare professional or registered dietitian to develop a personalized nutrition plan tailored to individual needs and preferences to ensure a smooth and successful recovery journey.

CHAPTER 3
BUILDING BLOCKS FOR COLLAGEN PRODUCTION

Collagen is a crucial protein that provides structure to various tissues in the body, including skin, tendons, ligaments, and muscles. It plays a vital role in maintaining skin elasticity, promoting wound healing, and supporting overall tissue integrity. Therefore, optimizing collagen production is essential, especially for individuals undergoing facelift surgery, as it can aid in the healing process and contribute to better surgical outcomes. Understanding the building blocks for collagen production and incorporating them into a post-surgery nutrition plan is paramount for facilitating recovery and promoting long-term wellness.

Essential Nutrients for Collagen Synthesis

Several key nutrients play integral roles in collagen synthesis within the body. These nutrients act as cofactors, enzymes, or structural components necessary for the production and maintenance of collagen fibers. Vitamin C stands out as a primary nutrient essential for collagen synthesis. It serves as a cofactor for the enzymes involved in collagen formation and helps stabilize the collagen molecule's structure. Including ample sources of vitamin C in the diet, such as citrus fruits, strawberries, bell peppers, and leafy greens, is crucial for supporting collagen production post-surgery.

Another vital nutrient for collagen synthesis is protein, particularly those rich in amino acids like glycine, proline, and hydroxyproline, which are abundant in collagen fibers. Incorporating high-quality protein sources such as lean meats, poultry, fish, eggs, dairy products, legumes, and tofu into the diet provides the necessary amino acids to support collagen formation and tissue repair. Additionally, consuming foods rich in sulfur, such as garlic, onions, cruciferous vegetables, and eggs, is beneficial as sulfur-containing amino acids like cysteine and methionine are essential for collagen synthesis.

Omega-3 fatty acids also play a role in collagen production by reducing inflammation and supporting skin health. Salmon, mackerel, sardines, flaxseeds, chia seeds, and walnuts are all great foods that are high in omega-3s. of omega-3s that can be included in a post-surgery nutrition plan to promote collagen synthesis and enhance healing.

Furthermore, micronutrients like copper, zinc, and manganese are involved in collagen metabolism and cross-linking, essential processes for collagen stability and functionality. These minerals can be obtained from a variety of foods, including nuts, seeds, whole grains, seafood, and legumes.

Incorporating a diverse array of nutrient-rich foods that provide essential vitamins, minerals, and amino acids is essential for supporting collagen synthesis and optimizing the healing process post-facelift surgery.

A well-rounded nutrition plan that prioritizes these key nutrients can contribute to improved wound healing, skin elasticity, and long-term tissue health.

Recipes Rich in Collagen-Boosting Ingredients

Creating meals that incorporate collagen-boosting ingredients is an effective way to support the body's natural healing processes post-facelift surgery. Including foods rich in vitamin C, protein, sulfur-containing amino acids, omega-3 fatty acids, and collagen-supportive minerals can enhance the nutritional value of meals and promote optimal collagen synthesis. Here are some recipes featuring collagen-boosting ingredients:

1. Citrus-Marinated Grilled Salmon: This recipe combines the omega-3 fatty acids found in salmon with vitamin C-rich citrus marinade to support collagen production and reduce inflammation. Marinate salmon fillets in a mixture of freshly squeezed lemon or orange juice, minced garlic, olive oil, and herbs like thyme or rosemary. Grill until cooked through and serve with a side of steamed broccoli and quinoa for a nutritious meal rich in collagen-boosting nutrients.

2. Bone Broth Vegetable Soup: Bone broth is a potent source of collagen, providing the body with essential amino acids and minerals necessary for collagen synthesis.

Simmer bones (such as chicken or beef bones) with vegetables like carrots, celery, onions, and garlic in water for several hours to extract the nutrients. Season with herbs and spices like turmeric, ginger, and parsley for added flavor and anti-inflammatory benefits. Enjoy this nourishing soup as a comforting meal post-surgery to promote healing and support tissue repair.

3. Greek Yogurt Parfait with Berries and Nuts: Greek yogurt is an excellent source of protein and calcium, which are essential for collagen synthesis and bone health. Put fresh berries (like raspberries, strawberries, or blueberries) on top of the Greek yoghurt and top with a sprinkle. of nuts and seeds (like almonds, walnuts, or chia seeds) for added texture and nutrient density.

Drizzle with a touch of honey or maple syrup for sweetness, if desired. This parfait makes for a satisfying and nutrient-rich breakfast or snack option to support post-surgery recovery and long-term wellness.

4. Quinoa Salad with Roasted Vegetables and Avocado: Quinoa is a complete protein containing all essential amino acids, making it an excellent addition to a collagen-boosting diet.

Toss cooked quinoa with roasted vegetables (such as bell peppers, zucchini, and cherry tomatoes) and diced avocado for a nourishing and flavorful salad. Drizzle with a homemade vinaigrette made from olive oil, lemon juice, garlic, and herbs for added antioxidant and anti-inflammatory benefits.

This vibrant salad provides a balanced mix of nutrients to support collagen synthesis and promote overall health.

5. Green Smoothie with Spinach and Kiwi: Leafy greens like spinach are rich in vitamin C and antioxidants that support collagen production and protect against oxidative stress. Blend fresh spinach with ripe kiwi, banana, and a splash of coconut water or almond milk for a refreshing and nutrient-dense smoothie. Add a scoop of protein powder or a dollop of Greek yogurt for an extra protein boost. Enjoy this green smoothie as a hydrating and revitalizing snack to fuel the body with essential nutrients post-surgery.

Incorporating these collagen-boosting recipes into a post-facelift surgery nutrition plan can provide the body with the necessary nutrients to support healing, promote tissue repair, and enhance long-term wellness.

By prioritizing foods rich in vitamin C, protein, omega-3 fatty acids, and collagen-supportive minerals, individuals can optimize the healing process and support overall tissue health for improved surgical outcomes.

CHAPTER 4
HYDRATION AND SKIN HEALTH

Hydration is a fundamental aspect of overall health and well-being, and its importance is especially pronounced in the context of skin health, particularly in the aftermath of facelift surgery. Understanding the pivotal role hydration plays in skin recovery can significantly aid individuals in optimizing their post-surgery nutrition plan. Adequate hydration is essential for maintaining the skin's elasticity, promoting collagen production, and facilitating the healing process. When the body is well-hydrated, it can efficiently transport essential nutrients to the skin cells, aiding in repair and regeneration. Additionally, proper hydration helps flush out toxins and waste products from the body, which can further support the healing process and promote a clear, radiant complexion.

The Role of Hydration in Skin Recovery

Post-surgery, the body undergoes a series of physiological processes aimed at repairing and rebuilding tissues damaged during the procedure. Hydration plays a crucial role in facilitating these processes, as it ensures that the body has an adequate supply of fluids to support cellular repair and regeneration.

Dehydration, on the other hand, can impair these processes, leading to delayed healing, increased inflammation, and compromised skin health. Moreover, dehydration can exacerbate common post-surgery side effects such as dryness, itching, and irritation, making it essential to prioritize hydration as part of the recovery process.

To maintain optimal hydration levels, it is recommended to consume a sufficient amount of water throughout the day. While individual hydration needs may vary based on factors such as body weight, activity level, and climate, a general guideline is to aim for at least eight glasses of water per day. However, individuals recovering from facelift surgery may need to increase their fluid intake to compensate for fluid loss during the healing process. Hydration should be a continuous effort, with small, frequent sips of water throughout the day rather than consuming large amounts at once. Additionally, incorporating hydrating foods such as fruits and vegetables into the diet can further support hydration levels and provide essential vitamins and minerals necessary for skin health.

Refreshing Beverages to Keep You Hydrated and Nourished

While water is undoubtedly the best choice for hydration, several other refreshing beverages can help keep you hydrated and nourished during the post-surgery recovery period. Herbal teas, such as chamomile or ginger tea, not only provide hydration but also offer soothing properties that can help alleviate post-surgery discomfort and promote relaxation.

Additionally, coconut water is an excellent natural source of electrolytes, making it an ideal choice for replenishing fluids and minerals lost during the recovery process.

Incorporating freshly squeezed juices into your diet can also be a flavorful way to boost hydration and provide essential nutrients. Opt for juices made from hydrating fruits such as watermelon, cucumber, and citrus fruits, which are rich in vitamins and antioxidants that support skin health and promote healing. Smoothies made with hydrating ingredients like leafy greens, berries, and yogurt can also be an excellent option for a nourishing and hydrating snack or meal replacement.

When selecting beverages during the recovery period, it's essential to avoid sugary drinks, caffeinated beverages, and alcohol, as these can have a dehydrating effect and may interfere with the body's healing processes. Instead, focus on hydrating beverages that provide essential nutrients and support overall health and well-being. By prioritizing hydration and incorporating refreshing beverages into your post-surgery nutrition plan, you can promote optimal skin recovery and long-term wellness.

CHAPTER 5
SUPERFOODS FOR SKIN REJUVENATION

When considering a comprehensive approach to skin rejuvenation, diet plays a crucial role alongside other treatments such as facelift surgery.

A balanced and nutritious diet can significantly aid in the healing process post-surgery, as well as contribute to long-term skin health and vitality. In this guide, we'll delve into the concept of a facelift surgery nutrition plan, focusing particularly on the inclusion of superfoods known for their skin-nourishing properties.

Introduction to Skin-Nourishing Superfoods

Superfoods are nutrient-rich foods that are particularly beneficial for health and well-being due to their high content of vitamins, minerals, antioxidants, and other essential nutrients. When it comes to skin health and rejuvenation, certain superfoods stand out for their ability to promote collagen production, fight inflammation, protect against oxidative stress, and enhance overall skin appearance.

Among the most notable superfoods for skin rejuvenation are berries such as blueberries, strawberries, and raspberries, which are packed with antioxidants that combat free radicals and promote collagen synthesis. A, C, and E can be found in large amounts in leafy veggies like spinach, kale, and Swiss chard. well as minerals like iron and magnesium, all of which are vital for skin health and regeneration.

Additionally, fatty fish like salmon, mackerel, and sardines are excellent sources of omega-3 fatty acids, which help maintain skin hydration, reduce inflammation, and support skin elasticity. Nuts and seeds, such as almonds, walnuts, flaxseeds, and chia seeds, provide essential fatty acids, vitamins, and minerals that contribute to skin nourishment and repair.

Other skin-nourishing superfoods include avocado, rich in healthy fats and vitamin E; tomatoes, abundant in lycopene, a powerful antioxidant; and green tea, known for its polyphenol content, which protects the skin from UV damage and promotes collagen synthesis.

Incorporating Superfoods into Delicious Meals

Incorporating superfoods into your diet doesn't have to be a daunting task; in fact, it can be both enjoyable and delicious. One effective way to incorporate these nutrient-packed foods is by incorporating them into various meals and recipes.

Starting the day with a nutritious breakfast is key, and options like a smoothie bowl made with berries, spinach, avocado, and a sprinkle of seeds can provide a powerhouse of skin-loving nutrients. Alternatively, oatmeal topped with fresh fruits, nuts, and a drizzle of honey offers a satisfying and nourishing start to the day.

For lunch and dinner, salads are an excellent way to pack in a variety of superfoods. A colorful salad featuring leafy greens, tomatoes, bell peppers, cucumber, avocado, and grilled salmon or tofu provides a well-rounded meal rich in vitamins, minerals, and healthy fats. Incorporating quinoa or lentils adds protein and fiber for sustained energy and satiety.

Snacks can also be an opportunity to boost your intake of superfoods. A handful of mixed nuts, a piece of fruit with almond butter, or a serving of Greek yogurt with berries and a sprinkle of seeds are all nutritious options that support skin health and overall well-being.

incorporating superfoods into your diet is an effective strategy for supporting skin rejuvenation, both during the post-surgery recovery period and in the long term.

By including a variety of nutrient-dense foods rich in antioxidants, vitamins, minerals, and healthy fats, you can nourish your skin from the inside out, promoting a radiant complexion and optimal skin health.

CHAPTER 6
MAINTAINING LONG-TERM RESULTS

Sustainable Nutrition Habits for Lasting Effects:

Achieving optimal results from facelift surgery goes beyond the operating table; it requires a commitment to long-term lifestyle choices, particularly in the realm of nutrition. Sustainable nutrition habits play a pivotal role in preserving the rejuvenated appearance attained through the surgical procedure. By understanding the significance of nutrient-rich foods, individuals can foster an environment conducive to healing, enhance skin health, and prolong the longevity of their facelift results.

Nutrition serves as the cornerstone of post-surgery recovery and maintenance. In the context of facelift surgery, where the skin undergoes significant trauma and subsequent healing, the body's nutritional needs are heightened.

Adequate intake of essential nutrients, including vitamins, minerals, protein, and antioxidants, is crucial for supporting tissue repair, collagen synthesis, and overall skin health. Moreover, a balanced diet contributes to immune function, reduces inflammation, and promotes cellular regeneration, all of which are imperative for optimal recovery and long-term results.

Following a facelift surgery, adhering to a well-rounded and nutrient-dense diet is essential for promoting healing, reducing inflammation, and optimizing long-term results. This comprehensive guide offers insights into crafting a post-surgery nutrition plan, featuring healing recipes, meal plans, and expert tips for sustained wellness.

Nutrient-Rich Foods:

Incorporating a variety of nutrient-rich foods into the post-surgery diet is paramount for supporting the body's healing process and maintaining skin health. Fresh fruits and vegetables, such as berries, leafy greens, citrus fruits, and bell peppers, provide an abundance of vitamins, minerals, and antioxidants essential for collagen production, tissue repair, and combating oxidative stress. Lean proteins, including poultry, fish, tofu, and legumes, supply the necessary building blocks for tissue regeneration and immune function. Whole grains, nuts, seeds, and healthy fats, such as avocados and olive oil, offer additional nutrients and promote skin hydration and elasticity.

Hydration:

Proper hydration is fundamental for post-surgery recovery and skin health. Adequate water intake helps flush out toxins, maintains skin hydration, and supports cellular function. Individuals recovering from facelift surgery should aim to consume at least eight glasses of water per day, and more if engaging in strenuous activities or experiencing increased fluid loss due to medications or environmental factors.

Meal Planning:

Structured meal planning can aid in adhering to a nutritious diet and ensuring constant intake of important nutrients. Planning meals ahead of time allows individuals to incorporate a range of nutrient-dense foods into their diet, balance macronutrient intake, and prevent reliance on processed or convenience foods that may delay healing and undermine long-term effects. Incorporating a varied range of colors, textures, and flavors into meals not only boosts nutritional content but also makes the dining experience more fun and rewarding.

Supplementation:

In some circumstances, supplements may be necessary to address specific nutritional deficiencies or promote the body's healing process post-surgery. Consulting with a healthcare practitioner or qualified dietitian can assist in identifying specific supplement needs based on characteristics such as age, health state, and dietary intake. Common supplements prescribed for post-surgery healing may include vitamin C, vitamin D, zinc, omega-3 fatty acids, and collagen peptides, among others.

Expert Tips:

In addition to adopting a nutrient-dense diet, numerous professional advice can further optimize post-surgery nutrition and enhance long-term effects. These tips include:

1. Prioritize Protein Intake: Protein is needed for tissue repair and wound healing. Incorporate lean sources of protein throughout each meal, such as grilled chicken, fish, tofu, or beans, to support healthy recovery and collagen synthesis.

2. Limit Sugar and Processed Foods: High-sugar and processed foods can worsen inflammation, hinder wound healing, and jeopardize skin health.

Minimize consumption of sugary snacks, refined carbohydrates, and processed foods, choosing instead for complete, unprocessed alternatives.

3. Focus on Anti-Inflammatory Foods: Incorporating anti-inflammatory foods, such as turmeric, ginger, garlic, and fatty fish rich in omega-3 fatty acids, can help reduce post-surgery inflammation, alleviate discomfort, and promote recovery.

4. Practice Mindful Eating: Mindful eating entails paying attention to hunger cues, relishing each meal, and eating carefully to promote digestion and nutritional absorption. Avoid distractions such as television or technological gadgets during meals, and focus on the sensory experience of eating.

5. Stay Consistent with Medications and Supplements: Adhering to prescribed medications and supplement regimens as suggested by healthcare providers is vital for supporting the

body's healing process and enhancing post-surgery recovery. Be sure to take medications and supplements at the appropriate times and doses to maximum efficacy.

By incorporating this professional advice into a comprehensive post-surgical nutrition plan, patients undergoing facelift surgery can promote maximum recovery, preserve skin health, and achieve long-lasting benefits.

With a commitment to sustainable eating practices and conscious dietary choices, individuals can boost their general well-being and enjoy the benefits of a rejuvenated appearance for years to come.

Recipes for Ongoing Skin Health Maintenance:

Following facelift surgery, maintaining skin health becomes a concern for individuals looking to retain the results of their procedure and encourage long-term wellness. Incorporating healthy dishes into the post-surgery diet can give critical nutrients, antioxidants, and moisture necessary for supporting skin health, boosting collagen formation, and decreasing indications of aging. From nutrient-packed smoothies to antioxidant-rich salads and collagen-boosting soups, these therapeutic dishes offer delicious and healthful solutions for continuous skin health maintenance.

Healing Smoothies:

Smoothies are a great method to combine many nutrients into one tasty and portable drink.

Adding foods like leafy greens, berries, avocado, Greek yogurt, nut butter, and avocado can provide you with an abundance of vitamins, minerals, antioxidants, and healthy fats that are vital for maintaining the health of your skin and accelerating the healing process after surgery.

Try making a nutrient-dense, hydrating smoothie using frozen berries, bananas, Greek yogurt, almond milk, spinach, and kale. This will nourish your body from the inside out.

Salads are a flexible, nutrient-dense choice that can help with skin health and the healing process after surgery. Salads can be enhanced by adding a variety of fruits, vegetables, nuts, seeds, lean proteins, and other colorful ingredients that are high in vitamins, minerals, antioxidants, and phytonutrients that are necessary for tissue repair, collagen formation, and inflammation reduction.

For a tasty and antioxidant-rich salad that promotes skin health and accelerates healing, try tossing together mixed greens, cherry tomatoes, cucumbers, bell peppers, avocado, walnuts, grilled chicken, and a drizzle of olive oil and balsamic vinegar.

Soups that Boost Collagen:

Soups are a soothing and nourishing food choice for people getting over a facelift. Including collagen-promoting nutrients-rich foods and beverages, such as bone broth, veggies, herbs, and spices, can help maintain skin health, encourage tissue regeneration, and improve healing after surgery. Try combining carrots, celery, onion, garlic, ginger, turmeric, and beef or chicken bone broth with spinach to make a tasty, collagen-boosting soup that supports maximum healing and feeds the body.

Drinks that Rehydrate:

It's critical to stay hydrated to support skin health and the healing process following surgery.

Fresh fruit, herbs, and spices can be added to water to improve hydration, offer vital nutrients, and give ordinary water a taste explosion. Slices of cucumber, lemon, lime, and mint can be added to water to create a pleasant and hydrating drink that benefits skin health and enhances general well-being.

People may provide their bodies with the vital nutrients, antioxidants, and water required to improve skin health, enhance collagen formation, and promote long-term benefits by adding these healing recipes into a post-surgery diet regimen. People may maximize their recuperation after surgery and take pleasure in the advantages of a refreshed appearance for years to come by committing to eating healthily and using pure substances.

CHAPTER 7
FEEDING THE SOUL AND THE BODY

Any surgical operation, including a facelift, requires a recovery process that goes beyond physical healing to include mental and emotional restoration. In this holistic approach to well-being, nutrition is crucial because it affects the body's capability to heal as well as the mind's ability to deal with the changes and difficulties that accompany surgery. In this in-depth guide to the best post-surgical diet for recently diagnosed patients having facelift surgery, we examine mindful eating techniques for holistic well-being as well as the psychological effects of nutrition on healing.

Nutrition's Psychological Effects on Healing

There is a close relationship between nutrition and mental health since the things we eat affect both our physical and emotional states.

During the healing phase following facelift surgery, patients may feel a variety of feelings, such as tension, anxiety, and dissatisfaction with their look. A more optimistic view and a reduction in negative emotions may be fostered by proper diet, which has a substantial impact on mood and cognitive function.

Studies have indicated that some nutrients are important for mental health and brain function. Omega-3 fatty acids, for instance, which are included in walnuts, flaxseeds, and fatty fish, have been connected to better mood and a lower risk of depression. Similarly, oxidative stress and inflammation in the brain, which can lead to mental health disorders, are fought off by meals high in antioxidants, like fruits, vegetables, and green tea.

Maintaining a healthy diet after surgery can also help patients feel more empowered and in charge of their lives, both of which are important for psychological health. Adhering to a regimented eating schedule that emphasizes nutrient-dense foods gives people a feeling of direction and control during a vulnerable time, fostering self-efficacy and resilience in the face of hardship.

Practices of Mindful Eating for Complete Wellbeing

Apart from emphasizing the nutritional value of food, mindful eating techniques can also improve the overall well-being of patients having facelift surgery. Observing the taste, texture, and scent of food as well as identifying signals of hunger and fullness are all part of mindful eating.

The capacity of mindful eating to develop a stronger bond between the mind and body by encouraging a greater awareness and appreciation of food is one of its main advantages. People can have a healthier, guilt-free relationship with eating by learning to appreciate every bite and adopting a nonjudgmental mindset towards food.

Additionally, being mindful during meals can assist people in identifying the emotional triggers that lead to overindulgence in food or unhealthy eating patterns, enabling them to respond to these triggers with greater expertise. Maladaptive eating behaviors are less common when people learn to deal with their emotions head-on rather than turning to food as a coping mechanism for stress or boredom.

Since the body can process and assimilate nutrients more easily when it is relaxed, incorporating mindfulness into mealtime practices can also help with digestion and nutritional absorption. People can optimize their digestive process, reducing discomfort and boosting general gastrointestinal health, by eating slowly and fully digesting their food.

People can begin incorporating mindful eating into their post-surgery diet plan by designating a certain time for meals, away from distractions like television or electronics. Before eating, they can also engage in mindful breathing exercises or meditation to develop a sense of presence and tranquility. Furthermore, monitoring eating habits and moods with a food journal can assist people in pinpointing areas for development and in making more thoughtful food choices.

optimal healing and long-term well-being following facelift surgery depend on feeding the body and mind. People can enhance their physical and mental well-being by adopting mindful eating practices into their daily routine and by being aware of the psychological effects of nutrition on recovery. By using a comprehensive nutritional strategy that includes therapeutic recipes, meal plans, and professional advice, people can set out on a path to improved internal and external health and vitality.

CONCLUSION

This thorough manual is an invaluable tool for anyone navigating the recuperation process following surgery, especially those who have had facelifts. Comprehending the complex relationship between diet and the healing process is essential since it can greatly impact an individual's recuperation process.

This guide has covered a wide range of nutrition-related topics, from long-term wellness plans to pre-surgery preparation. We have discussed the significance of eating foods high in nutrients to prime the body for surgery and have included recipes for detoxing and cleansing to maximize the time leading up to the procedure.

We've underlined the importance of addressing certain nutritional demands to promote healing throughout the crucial post-surgery recovery phase, including liquid and soft food diets. We've also looked at anti-inflammatory recipes that are meant to lessen bruises and swelling so that healing goes more smoothly.

It's critical to comprehend the fundamental components of collagen synthesis to support skin health following surgery. To encourage the best possible healing, we've compiled recipes full of collagen-boosting foods and insights into these nutrients.

We've talked about the importance of hydration for skin recovery as well as several cool drink choices to keep you nourished and hydrated during the process.

In addition, we've covered skin-nourishing superfoods and shown you how to combine them into delectable dishes to revitalize and nourish your skin from the inside out.

To ensure that the advantages of the procedure are optimized over time, we have included recipes and defined sustainable eating practices for long-term, sustained outcomes.

We've now covered the psychological effects of diet on recovery and mindful eating strategies, highlighting the importance of overall wellness for the body and mind.

Essentially, this guide helps people optimize their post-surgery recovery journey and attain long-lasting effects by providing expert suggestions and insights for long-term wellness in addition to healing recipes and meal plans.